Contents

Introduction

Why is it that every time you turn on the TV or open a newspaper these days there will probably be a story about food? It is interesting that the stories in question are very rarely positive. We hear or read about food poisoning levels from E. coli or salmonella, the use of pesticides or antibiotics in animals, BSE, genetically modified (GM) foods – the list goes on and on.

So, what do we do – take precautions by not eating a particular product, or choose not to believe the information and carry on as before? Given that we all have to eat, it is hard to ignore the number of foods which seem to be suspect at any given time. There also seems to be a great deal of confusion about what is the 'truth'. Where one person may say that a particular foodstuff is 'safe', there is always one or more to say that there is a risk to us from eating it. It is not surprising that a lot of people get so frustrated that they ignore food safety information for the simple reason that 'if you believed everything you read or heard, you wouldn't eat anything'.

How do you react when you hear or read about food safety on the news or in the papers? Are you concerned? Do you stop eating the product in question? Do you think differently depending on what kind of food is at risk, or what type of food scare is being highlighted? Do you think more about the risks from BSE-infected meat or the threat of being poisoned from an egg or vice versa? Have you stopped to look at the packets of food products to see if there are any GM ingredients there? If not, why not? Think about it – certainly none of us think about what we are eating all of the time, but there are times when you can't help but notice that food safety is a big political issue. It is at these times that people potentially take stock of what they eat and decide whether to believe the information they are hearing or reading and whether to carry on as before or make changes to eating habits. The question here is what factors determine what people will do.

It is undoubtedly the case that food has become an important political and public issue. As agriculture develops and new technologies are brought onto the market, questions are being asked about how our food is produced and how safe it is. While it is easy to blame a lot of food 'scares' on media sensationalism (as though the problem doesn't really exist outside of a newspaper), it is clear that there are issues which governments, pressure groups and the food industry are having to deal with in a modern world of intensified food production. As such, we, as consumers, need to look at different levels of the debate and at key factors which may help to explain why certain issues become high profile. This book will look behind front-page headlines at how certain stories develop and the role played by government bodies, pressure groups, scientists, professional groups and consumers in determining the seriousness of different food safety issues.

The Growth
of Interest in Food Safety

Interest in food safety has been helped along by a number of factors. Three of the main influences have been the role played by government in legislating and implementing food safety measures, the development of pressure groups actively campaigning to ensure that safety levels of foodstuffs are acceptable, and the growth of interest by the mass media in Britain.

Until recently, the major public concern has been whether enough food is available. As food systems developed capacities to provide increasingly stable supplies of adequate food, people could focus more on food's qualitative aspects. Questions of quantity became replaced with concerns about ensuring the best possible food supply for health, leading to questions such as: Are pesticides and additives dangerous? What foods promote longevity? Does biotechnology create a healthier or more dangerous food supply?…When people have more choices and increasing opportunities to make their grievances known, they are also more likely to view the quality of their food as problematic.

Eating Agendas: Food and Nutrition as Social Problems by D. Maurer and J. Sobal (eds.), New York, Aldine de Gruyter, 1995

The mass media are blamed constantly for causing food 'scares'; they are regarded as being sensationalist and irresponsible by highlighting issues, and criticized for getting their facts wrong. The most frequent criticism of the news media is that they blow up otherwise inconsequential problems out of all proportion. While this may be the case on some occasions (and more so for certain parts of the media), it is important to understand that a number of different people and institutions are involved in attempting to define whether any particular foodstuff is either 'safe' or 'unsafe'.

The debates concerning food safety in Britain arose at a particular time in history and for particular reasons which must be addressed in order to obtain a clearer understanding of why they happened. This book will examine the factors which led to the emergence of concerns over certain food safety issues in Britain. Using a case-study approach it will look at some of the prominent 'scares' which have been highlighted in the British media. These will include BSE, salmonella and GM foods (and with reference to both E. coli and listeriosis). While these are very different types of food safety issue, there is a sense in which, as you will see, they are connected. We will look at the high-profile crisis around salmonella in eggs in 1988 which caused a drop in sales of up to 50 per cent. The next chapter seeks to go behind the media headlines to explain why 'mad cow' disease became one of the biggest food safety 'scares' in Britain, said to have cost almost £5 billion to sort out. Following on from BSE we will see how the issue of GM food has become so high profile and what arguments are being put forward by different people claiming that these products are either 'safe' or 'unsafe' for human health.

The role of the government

One of the key factors which has characterized a number of food scares has been the role of government in relation to food safety. There have been cases of apparent divisions between the different departments (as with salmonella), alleged secrecy among government departments (as with listeria and BSE), and potential failures in properly stringent legislative powers (as with E. coli), all of which have meant, in certain circumstances, that food safety becomes 'news'. The role of government is therefore central to the nature of high-profile food safety issues.

As we shall see later, divisions between government departments can cause major problems in relation to food safety. Government secrecy can also be a factor in a number of key food safety issues. The idea that governments might 'cover up' information that might affect our health means that these issues (if they become public) will undoubtedly be very high profile. If journalists are given no information from government on a particular issue, they will commonly call on other sources such as non-government scientists or pressure groups to find out what is 'really' going on. This was undoubtedly the case with BSE.

Perceived cover-ups were also at the centre of the 'scare' around listeria which began in earnest in 1989 when a TV programme (*This Week*, Thames TV, 24 January 1989) stated that a high percentage of cook-chilled food was infected with listeria. As sales dropped, food producers demanded that the government issue guidelines on cooking, storage and hygiene requirements when dealing with cook-chill. Yet in 1987/8, when the government had already been warned about the dangers of listeria from a number of foods such as chicken, cook-chill and soft cheese, they were still deciding how to handle the rise in cases. Reports from other countries pointed to a huge epidemic. In 1985 soft cheese infected with listeria killed sixty people in America. In Switzerland in 1987 a local soft cheese caused five deaths. It became clear that other countries were having a major problem with listeria and the common foodstuffs blamed were soft cheeses, pâtés, chicken dishes and cook-chill. It was also known that listeria could cause miscarriages, stillbirths and serious illnesses in newborn babies. In 1988 the World Health Organization (WHO) had issued information to governments that pregnant women and unborn children were at risk and urged governments to make the public aware of the dangers. Still it took the British government until 1989 to offer advice, two years after they had become aware of the danger. By that time it was reported that at least 26 unborn children and others had suffered serious illnesses. So, why weren't pregnant women warned?

Following in the wake of salmonella, listeria was seen as another potentially huge food issue. The relevant government departments did not want another food 'scare' on their hands. There were also the interests of the producers to take into consideration. If warnings were given then a large number of businesses would be affected (sales of eggs had been badly hit by the salmonella affair). So, the government played down the risks of listeria. But the birth of a child with cerebral palsy in January 1989 forced government officials to realize that they could no longer keep quiet. The Chief Medical Officer issued a warning of the risks of listeria to pregnant women.

Listeria

Listeria can be found in many places – in soil, sewage, silage, dust, water and in many domestic and wild animals. The bacterium does not change the taste or the smell of contaminated food and you can be unaware of it.

People infected with listeria may display flu-like symptoms, often with fever and chills. Fatigue, nausea, vomiting, diarrhoea, severe headaches and stiff necks are also other symptoms. The disease primarily affects pregnant women, new-borns, people with weakened immune systems and those over sixty.

How can listeria be prevented?
- thoroughly cook beef, pork, poultry and other raw food from animal sources;
- wash raw vegetables thoroughly before eating;
- keep uncooked meats separate from vegetables, cooked foods and ready-to-eat foods;
- avoid raw milk or foods made from raw milk.

Pregnant woman and others at high risk should also:
- avoid soft cheeses such as Brie or Camembert;
- heat left-over food or ready-to-eat food until steaming hot before eating.

Another issue relating to the role of government is the perceived inadequacy of particular food safety regulations concerning potential failures in properly using legislative powers. It is clear from some food safety cases that sometimes laws are not good enough to deal with the problem at hand. If, for example, there is an outbreak of a particular food poisoning epidemic, is it always appropriate to follow the same procedures?

E. coli

E. coli is a bacteria that normally lives in the intestines of humans and animals. Although most strains of this bacteria are harmless, several are known to produce toxins that can cause diarrhoea. One particular E. coli strain called 0157:H7 can cause severe diarrhoea and kidney damage.

People infected can develop a range of symptoms. Some infected people may have mild diarrhoea or no symptoms at all. Most identified cases develop severe diarrhoea and abdominal cramps.

How can E. coli be prevented?

- always wash fresh fruits and vegetables thoroughly before eating;
- always clean surfaces that have come into contact with raw meat before any other item is placed on that surface;
- always wash hands thoroughly after handling raw meat and before handling any other utensil or food item;
- always cook meat until the juices run absolutely clear;
- don't buy any food that smells bad or fruits and vegetables that are bruised or shrivelled;
- keep meats separate from produce;
- discard cut produce if it has been out of the refrigerator for four hours or more;
- do not eat undercooked hamburger or other ground beef products;
- drink only pasteurized milk and milk products.

Can you treat an outbreak of salmonella, for example, in the same way as an outbreak of E. coli 0157, a potentially more lethal and newer organism? It is these types of questions that are asked all the time by public health officials attempting to contain food poisoning outbreaks. A look at what happened in a 1996 outbreak of E. coli 0157 in Scotland might highlight some of the problems of legislation and regulation.

'If one was to set out and design a nasty food poisoning bug you'd come up with E. coli 0157, not just because it can attack people and cause very serious damage and maybe even kill them, but it spreads very easily too. We only need to eat perhaps as few as ten actual bacteria, and millions and millions are needed to cover the head of a pin. You only need to eat a very small number to get infected and perhaps develop all these nasty consequences.'

Professor Hugh Pennington, interviewed on *Outbreak*, BBC2, 15 April 1998

In November 1996, in Lanarkshire, Scotland, a number of people began to fall ill. In a short space of time tests showed that the organism causing their illness was E. coli 0157. By the end of what was to become the world's biggest outbreak of E. coli 0157, twenty people were dead and over 500 had been infected. The problem was that while there are a large number of E. coli bacteria (most of which are benign), the 0157 strain has mutated into a toxic strain. It has been estimated that since its discovery in the 1980s it has infected about 40,000 people. It is interesting that although E. coli 0157 is such a potentially lethal bacterium, probably very few people knew about it before the huge outbreak in Lanarkshire. Why this was the case remains unclear. Certainly it is clear that there were real concerns from certain quarters much earlier on. As far back as 1991 the Chief Medical Officer had issued advice on cooking beefburgers.

While E. coli may have been rare, the number of cases was clearly rising. Outbreaks had occurred in a number of countries, including America, Japan and Scotland. By 1995 concern was being raised by health officials who claimed that the very real dangers of

Following an outbreak of a rare form of food poisoning, caused by the organism *Escherichia coli* 0157 (E. coli 0157), Sir Donald Acheson, Chief Medical Officer, issued advice on 14 February to everyone who cooks beefburgers to make sure they are thoroughly cooked right through. E-coli 0157 organisms are heat sensitive and can be readily destroyed by proper cooking. Sir Donald's advice applies equally to other similar minced meat products.
MAFF Food Safety Directorate Information, Bulletin No.10, February 1991

E. coli were going unheeded. In that year there were 247 cases in Scotland alone. It was suggested that E. coli was not a political priority, and therefore not a research priority, because it was not a health problem in animals.

The main issue surrounding the Lanarkshire E. coli outbreak centred on how the episode had been handled – had enough been done to ensure that the infection was stopped as quickly as possible? The Lanarkshire Health Authority had been alerted and the Environmental Health Office (EHO) brought in to help stem any potential epidemic. Their main priority was to isolate the source of the outbreak and remove any potentially contaminated food from the food chain. Once the source of the outbreak had been isolated to one particular butcher's shop, officials had a choice of action they could take. They could ask the butcher to voluntarily stop selling potentially infected meat, seize meats from his establishment or immediately close the shop. While the simplest course of action may seem to be to close any potentially infected premises down completely, a number of considerations were taken into account which meant that this was not done as quickly as it could have been. Firstly, there was the issue of balancing public health interests with that of the risks to the business. Secondly, health officials had to keep in mind that they could be sued if they were wrong. In 1995 a farmer was ordered not to sell his Lanark Blue cheese in case it was contaminated with listeria. The case went to court and the farmer was paid compensation. So, potentially out of date legislation (which offered choices to businesses) and financial considerations may have played a part in this outbreak.

> Outbreaks of E. coli were not a political priority. Not until the death toll for the outbreak in Wishaw [Lanarkshire] began to climb into double figures. But the evidence that something was going very wrong was there to be seen. It was there in the sad shape of children with kidney failure and brain damage. It was there in the growing number of elderly people stricken by the bug. It was there for all official sources to see in the figures produced every year for the government. Still the warnings went unheeded.
>
> Margaret Vaughan, *The Herald*, 8 February 1997

What actually happened was that officials visited the butcher and he agreed voluntarily to withdraw all cooked meats from sale. This decision was to have wide-ranging effects. Firstly, other foodstuffs remained on sale (for example, minced meat products, pies and sandwiches), which did not safely take into account the risks of cross-contamination. It was also alleged that cooked meats left the premises after the butcher had been told to stop selling them. The business at the centre of the scandal was also known to supply a number of other establishments. MPs became critical of the fact that a list of these establishments had not been handed over. Questions were asked about whether the interests of business and profits were being put before those of public health. But the fact was that the health officials dealing with the outbreak were apparently forbidden by law to hand out a list unless they knew that it was complete. The E. coli outbreak certainly raised questions about the power of contemporary food safety laws. Had a list been volunteered earlier and the butcher's shop closed down even one day sooner, perhaps a large number of people would not have been infected with a potentially lethal bacterium.

The role of pressure groups

In the past 15–20 years there has been an ever-increasing interest in more general food issues. Food has become international as we are exposed to foods from different cultures. In addition, there has been an increasing interest in both moral and ethical aspects of food production, seen through the development of, for example, vegetarianism or animal rights activism. These perspectives on food did not simply come along. There has been a history of campaigning groups who have worked to raise public awareness and concern about a number of aspects of food. The consumer movement developed in the 1970s, while in the 1980s campaigning groups such as the London Food Commission, National Food Alliance, Chicken Lib and the Farm Animal Welfare Network were set up to look into and attempt to change different aspects of the food production system. More recently, organizations such as Greenpeace and English Nature have become prominent because of their role in the debate about GM food and crops. The role of pressure groups has become ever more important, particularly since the late 1980s when government was perceived as being less trustworthy in relation to food safety. While these groups actively seek membership and produce bulletins, magazines etc., one of the main reasons they have become so high profile is because of their relationship with the mass media. As there have been so many instances where either the government or members of the food industry will not speak to the media, pressure groups have begun to fill the role of 'experts' as well as highlighting their own causes and campaigns.

The role of the media

There has not always been the avid interest there is now in food safety issues within the mainstream media. If you looked at newspapers or television in the 1970s, for example, you would not find anything like the level of coverage we now experience. This was because at that time food writing was clearly linked with cookery and seen as a 'women's issue'. It has also been suggested that the relationship between many journalists and the food industry might have been a little too close, so that many problems within the industries may not have been widely written about. But as with the growth of consumer and environmental politics in relation to food, mass media coverage has expanded to the point where there are food and consumer correspondents in a number of national newspapers and television news programmes, as well as a growing number of food-related shows and cookery programmes.

> Across the industrialised world people's interest in their own food has become intense. Cookbooks are reported to occupy a huge share of non-fiction sales. Elaborate television programmes on food are more numerous than ever; series that are game shows as well as cookery demonstrations, or travellers' tales of exotic ways of life as much as of unfamiliar cuisines. Full pages devoted to good eating and dining out are more firmly established in broadsheet newspapers, never mind whole magazines in glossy full colour.
> (*The Nation's Diet* by Anne Murcott, Longman, 1998)

With the growing interest in food within the media has come a growing interest in food safety and the politics of food. Still the most frequent criticism of the mass media is that they are sensationalist, making huge issues out of things that are not really important. But this is not always the case and we need to look a little at why some food safety issues might be more prone to media treatment than others. In other words, we need a basic understanding of how the media might work in relation to food 'scares'.

It is clear that news values may often produce coverage which is out of kilter with the needs and desires of government, industry or pressure group strategies. News values are oriented to maximizing audiences. Demands within the mass media for high-profile news (such as new information on food safety or food 'scares') may often produce coverage which does not necessarily fit with the needs of government, industry or pressure groups.

As we have already seen, the role of government is an important factor in the emergence of food 'scares'.

If an issue is seen to be politically 'hot' (like divisions within departments or governments being seen to 'cover up' information) then it will become a high-profile media story. This happened with all of the major food 'scares', but at the same time major stories can quite quickly disappear. Within the mass media it is controversy, political disagreements or failures of government that will keep a story in the news. If there is seen to be a resolution to the problem then it will be removed from the front pages of the newspapers.

For example, salmonella was one of the biggest food 'scares' of the decade, and yet it was removed from the front pages once Edwina Currie had resigned and a compensation package had been agreed; there was virtually no media coverage of BSE between 1992 and 1996 once European bans on British beef had been lifted; and since new regulations concerning E. coli were recommended, media coverage of E. coli 0157 has decreased even though there have since been more than 36 new outbreaks in Britain with over 1,600 reported cases.

No longer a political issue in which the guilty perpetrators can be identified, such a story also becomes difficult to run on the front page, especially for a mass market newspaper, because the guilty in this case are the newspapers' own consumers. Another reason for this lack of attention to food issues in general is that food and health are still regarded as 'soft' news, as more properly the concern of women, unless they become 'political' or pertain to scientific advances. Very early on in the salmonella affair the major issues being discussed were not how many chickens might be infected but how consumers (and specifically women) could cook and store eggs properly.

But some 'scares' do last longer than others. Although there was little coverage of BSE from 1992 to 1996, it was clear that because the issue of human transmission was unresolved, BSE could still periodically reappear on the front pages of the press. It is the very uncertainty about BSE that made it a continuing story, although its impact on human health is, so far as is known, inconsequential. This is, of course, quite different from the relationship between the media and *Salmonella Enteritidis*. Salmonella has a much greater known impact on human health and has continued to rise since 1988.

The story of food safety as a public issue in Britain illustrates the importance of the different parts that organizations play in helping to discourage or encourage debate on food safety issues. It is certainly the case that the most recent food safety 'scares' arose at a particular juncture in history for particular reasons. We will now move on to look at some of them in more detail.

Salmonella in Eggs

On 3 December 1988 the Junior Health Minister, Edwina Currie, told ITN:

> We do warn people now that most of the egg production of this country, sadly, is now infected with salmonella. If, however, they've used a good source of eggs, a good shop that they know, and they're content, then there seems no reason for them to stop. But we would advise against using raw egg – mayonnaise and dressings and Bloody Marys and that sort of thing. They are not a good idea anymore.

ITN News, 3 December 1988

Her remarks, broadcast on the news that evening, triggered one of the biggest food safety crises in post-war Britain. Within days egg sales had fallen by up to 50 per cent (Commons Agriculture Committee, 1990) and the egg industry was in disarray.

To understand why salmonella in eggs came upon the public scene it is necessary to explore a number of issues.

Salmonella

There are several types of salmonella infection, caused by inadequate cooking or contamination of cooked foods by bacteria from raw food. The main sources are raw meat and chicken, eggs and raw milk.

The symptoms are abdominal pain, diarrhoea, nausea, vomiting and fever. However, for people who are more vulnerable such as young children or the elderly, salmonella can cause serious problems such as meningitis or blood infections.

How can salmonella be prevented?

1. Always treat raw poultry, beef and pork as if they were contaminated and handle accordingly:
- wrap fresh meats in plastic bags at the market to prevent blood from dripping on other foods;
- refrigerate foods promptly, minimize holding at room temperature;
- wash cutting boards and counters used for preparation immediately after use to prevent cross contamination with other foods;
- avoid eating raw or undercooked meats;
- ensure that the correct internal cooking temperature is reached particularly when using a microwave.

2. Avoid eating raw eggs or undercooked foods containing raw eggs.

3. Avoid using raw milk.

4. Encourage careful handwashing before and after food preparation.

5. Make sure children, particularly those who handle pets, attend to handwashing.

Background

The salmonella in eggs incident did not happen by chance. There were a number of factors which came together to determine the widespread reaction to Edwina Currie's statement. Historically, changes in food production techniques and safety regulations had been occurring in Britain since the 1970s. Decisions on matters of food safety and hygiene were split between the Ministry of Agriculture, Fisheries and Food (MAFF) and the Department of Health (DoH). But food policy formation was affected when a number of issues appeared with which the departments had not previously had to deal. The interests of the farming community were less important than they had been in the post-war years, with the move to overproduction and with budgetary controls within the European Community. Added to this was the fact that with adequate supplies the notion of provision became less important than a newly acquired interest in healthier eating. The notion of health, the link between diet and disease, and the growth of food production technologies were all new issues in the food policy arena. The DoH accepted these new responsibilities by taking positions on food and health that were in opposition to MAFF. By the time that salmonella in eggs occurred there was no single decision-making centre dealing with new problems but two main bodies attempting to define their own responsibilities.

This oppositional situation was firmly in place in 1988 when reports of the existence of a virulent strain of *Salmonella Enteritidis* named Phage Type 4 (PT4) began to appear. While it was well known in some quarters, the issue of salmonella in chickens did not become one of political conflict. The view of politicians and civil servants was that salmonella in chickens was unavoidable and therefore the onus for prevention of poisoning was on the consumer rather than the farmer or the government. The new element brought in with the PT4 strain was whether eggs themselves were now being infected. The egg industry itself, it seems, felt that it had little reason to worry as it saw itself protected under the then government's historical 'laissez-faire' attitude to food policy and its ethos that health was related to individual choice. Also, had *Salmonella Enteritidis* been seen to physically affect poultry, the egg industry might have been less lax in its attitude to the increasing infection rates, but because it did not cause apparent infections in birds it was not deemed to be economically important to the industry.

The egg industry was already in some trouble because sales were in decline. Although eggs had been seen as part of a healthy and nutritious diet, their appeal had been waning for at least a decade. In 1990 Mintel reported a decline of 20 per cent in household consumption in that period because of what they called 'the evolution of eating habits'. Public awareness of the importance of healthy eating had already been well established, with government and medical campaigns as part of a drive to cut heart disease rates.

The emergence of the problem

The emergence into the public sphere of *Salmonella Enteritidis* as a potential health threat reflected the political stance being taken on its existence and on the treatment of other food risks. Throughout 1988 media coverage of food-borne risks had been varied, if not remarkably extensive: salmonella in pepperoni sticks, beansprouts and frozen or chilled chicken, paratyphoid from frozen curry meals, meningitis from Greek goat's cheese, listeria in pre-packed salads and cheese. Added to this were the more readily recognizable stories about outbreaks in, for example, restaurants, takeaways, hospitals, overseas holiday resorts and one in the House of Lords (May 1988). From January to the end of November 1988 there were a total of 263 national press and TV stories about these issues. 74 per cent of the stories were framed around individual consumers' and food outlets' hygiene and cooking practices.

The issue became relevant in policy circles because the number of cases of *Salmonella Enteritidis* reported in England and Wales had increased between 1981 (1,087) and 1987 (4,962). By the end of 1988 over 12,522 cases had been reported, a third of all known salmonella cases. *Salmonella Enteritidis* had first come to light with the publication of research by the American Centers for Disease Control (CDC) in April 1988. The CDC study claimed that salmonella was occurring in eggs, not only on contaminated eggshells but within the eggs themselves. The advice from the US was that, for complete safety from salmonella food poisoning, eggs should be boiled for a minimum of seven minutes, poached for five, or fried for three minutes on each side. This view was met with scepticism on the part of British health experts who claimed that the particular strain of salmonella in question, *Salmonella Enteritidis PT4*, was not commonly found in eggs in Britain. According to one DoH spokesman, 'there was no reason for any new advice about preparing eggs and chicken, beyond observing normal hygiene and ensuring both are thoroughly cooked' (*The Times*, 16 April 1988). But enough concern was felt for DoH and MAFF to set up a joint government working party to investigate the rise in cases. In August 1988 DoH issued a warning to hospitals about the risk of eating raw eggs (but not to the public and producers until November). Figures released by the Department, based on data from the Public Health Laboratory Service, showed that some 21 cases of salmonella in 1988 had been linked to eggs (*The Guardian,* 27 August 1988). More evidence of the problems with *Salmonella Enteritidis* appeared in a *Lancet* paper in September 1988. Then on 2 December 1988 Plymouth Health Authority took action and banned eggs from all of their hospitals. It was at this point that Edwina Currie made the issue public.

Instantly, a number of different interest groups, namely DoH, MAFF and the egg industry, were forced to become involved in an issue of public concern that they were not ready to handle. What Edwina Currie had unleashed, however unintentionally, was a number of problems associated with drawing public attention

1. 'In admitting that they have a problem with salmonella infection in the egg production industry, the Ministry of Agriculture, Fisheries and Food claim the actual rate of infection is very small indeed.'

2. 'The Department of Health, in reinforcing its warning about eating raw egg in any form, is advising everyone to ensure that all eggs are cooked until the yolk and white are hard. This advice is particularly important for those who are ill, pregnant women, the elderly and children.'

3. 'The United Kingdom Egg Producers Association labelled as a "load of rubbish" the claim about the extent of salmonella infection.'
ITN News, 3 December 1988

to a potential health risk which cuts across commercial interests. A number of very different positions were taken on this issue, as is clear from TV news on 3 December following Currie's statement.

Advice to consumers from the DoH was that, while eggs were a public health problem, individual eggs were unlikely to be infected. Precautions to be taken included stopping eating raw eggs or foods made with raw egg. While it was admitted that there was a risk, it was seen as an 'acceptable' risk for healthy people to eat soft eggs. Those deemed vulnerable (i.e. the elderly, young children, pregnant women and those with lowered immunity levels) were advised to eat eggs that had been cooked until they were hard.

The egg production industry demanded that something be done to restore public confidence in eggs, claiming that the minister's remarks were costing them £5 million per week and that the threat of bankruptcy loomed as many producers began to lose orders. The issue of blame became paramount. While it was a mark of government concern that a new voluntary code of practice for the egg industry was to be introduced, in the early stages of what would become known as the 'eggs crisis' blame was firmly put in the lap of the minister who had brought the issue to light. MAFF blamed Edwina Currie, claiming that she had been 'factually incorrect' in her statement which had been made without consulting them. The egg producers threatened legal action against Edwina Currie and demanded a full retraction and/or her resignation for the damage she had done to the industry. But Currie refused to retract her words and was eventually forced to resign two weeks after making her statement, following immense pressure.

Government action

With awareness raised the government had to respond very quickly to the problem. A Committee was set up to investigate the salmonella affair. In addition, a damage limitation strategy was necessary as the main protagonists were at pains to ensure that public confidence in eggs was restored. Agriculture Minister John MacGregor's department announced they would give half a million pounds to instigate a government advertising campaign to counter the scare. But a row developed as neither department could agree on how the advert should be worded. MAFF wanted it to say that eggs were safe to eat, but the DoH would not agree to such complete assurances of safety. The phrasing was finally agreed and a 200-word statement appeared which included the interests of both departments. It was generally criticized by the egg industry as being no more than a 'health warning' because it offered information on how to cook eggs 'safely'. With a national average drop of 60 per cent in sales, a surplus of 20 million unused eggs daily, 100,000 chickens being killed and the threat of job losses, the industry demanded compensation. The government announced a £19 million package on 19 December but still no answers were given about the actual safety of eggs. It seemed that the scientific experts were as divided as the politicians over the extent of the salmonella problem in eggs themselves. In the end it was left to the Chief Medical Officer to admit to the underlying uncertainties by saying that, while Britain was suffering an 'epidemic' increase of *Salmonella Enteritidis,* there was no clear scientific evidence to say that eggs were infected.

With Edwina Currie's resignation and the compensation package offered to the producers, the political battle moved inside Whitehall and out of the public gaze. The affair might not have resurfaced but for media reporting in January 1989 of the Commons Agriculture Committee's investigation which gave the public a chance to hear the full story. The debates around *Salmonella Enteritidis* were reopened as representatives of MAFF, DoH and the egg industry went to the committee armed with statistics which appeared to support their differing viewpoints. Contradictory evidence abounded but all parties seemed to agree on the fact that what Edwina Currie had said was wrong. The public profile of these proceedings was also heightened by Edwina Currie's refusal to appear before the committee to give evidence. Following three letters to her she eventually agreed to appear. She did not retract her statement and certainly did nothing to help clear up the question of the safety of eggs, saying that she had nothing new to add to the investigation. In fact, it was in an interview on Channel 4's documentary programme *Dispatches* on 25 October 1989 that Mrs Currie said, for the first time, not that she had been wrong, but rather that she had 'got the words wrong'. Up to this point she had refused to withdraw the remark 'most of the egg production', but she now claimed that she did not intend to say 'most eggs'; she should have said 'many' or 'some' or 'a few'. Almost nine months after the initial statement, it seemed that still no one knew the precise answer.

While the committee collected evidence, food safety was undoubtedly high on the political and media agendas. The end of *Salmonella Enteritidis* as a high-profile public issue came with the publication of the Agriculture Select Committee's report on the affair in February 1989. The report criticized Edwina Currie but also put the affair down to a failure of government. They recommended that to deal with the complexity of the salmonella problem there needed to be more research and resources, the development of procedures for tracing food outbreaks, compensation for the slaughter of infected breeding and laying flocks, assurances that catering establishments used pasteurized eggs in all uncooked egg dishes, and a properly funded campaign to promote better hygiene in the home.

Following this, media interest in the story dissipated as a resolution to the affair was seen to have been reached, both at the political level and with the constant reminders to consumers of how to cook eggs 'properly'. Egg sales also began to rise again slowly and were up to around 75 per cent of earlier levels by early 1989 (Mintel, 1990). From 244 newspaper stories in January 1989, there were only twenty in the whole of April of that year. The issue was never again to enjoy such a high profile in the British media. Interestingly, while media interest has undoubtedly diminished since 1988/9, in 1997, according to Public Health Laboratory figures, cases of *Salmonella Enteritidis* were higher than they were in 1988, accounting for 71 per cent (22,806) of all *Salmonella* cases reported, while the PT4 strain accounted for 47 per cent of all *Enteritidis* cases (Public Health Laboratory Service, 1997).

It is also interesting to note that the same warning about how to cook eggs was broadcast on TV news programmes on 9 April 1998 with nothing like the same impact it had caused ten years before. Why was this the case? There is a sense in which the salmonella affair was less a food 'scare' and more a political 'scare'. What seemed to be most important at the time was the role played by both the DoH and MAFF and the battle played out to assess who should be handling food safety.

Conclusion

The salmonella in eggs affair in Britain was both a political and a historical problem. The reason why agriculture had historically been linked to food was to increase food production. Farmers were given responsibility for this and food output was the prime objective. But problems arose when these objectives had been satisfied and questions were being asked about whether one minister could properly represent both producers and consumers. The professional rivalries of the two departments involved were highlighted and for once the British public was privy to the nature of interdepartmental disputes.

The salmonella affair did lead to the restructuring of food laws in Britain with the announcement of a new food safety bill in March 1990. With calls from the opposition parties for a Consumer Ministry separate from MAFF, instead there was introduced a 'Food Minister' responsible for food safety and a Food Safety Directorate within MAFF itself. For the first time, responsibility for food production and safety were separated as the government attempted to be seen to be publicly accountable.

So, was Edwina Currie correct? In relation to egg production there was undoubtedly a problem with salmonella in flocks, which was admitted. But there was no clear scientific evidence about whether individual eggs were infected and to what extent. The Agriculture Select Committee report stated that:

Background

Since the drive for increased food output during World War Two, cattle have been fed cheap high-protein cattle-feed (abattoir waste, including sheep's brains processed into meal) to maximize production of beef bulk, calves and milk. In the late 1970s rules regarding how rendering plants were run changed. Feed-renderers altered their methods in order to cut costs, including a switch from high-heat batch production which was used to help kill off agents such as scrapie from sheep waste.

In April 1985 a vet was called out to see a cow in Ashford, Kent. The animal was panicky and aggressive, and began drooling and falling over. The vet assumed the cause was a brain tumour, put the animal down and thought nothing more of it. That is, until he was called back to the same farm to see a second cow with the same symptoms. More cases followed. He discovered that the brains of the animals had a spongy texture similar to those of sheep infected with scrapie. He called in the local MAFF vet, and in November 1986 the Central Veterinary Laboratory (CVL) in Surrey confirmed what was thought to be the world's first case of spongiform brain disease in cattle.

A number of factors influenced the rise of BSE as an important public issue. The main issues involve the role of government and scientific uncertainty surrounding a new disease.

Government response

MAFF took complete control over all aspects of BSE. It was not until June 1986 (seven months after the first diagnosis) that MAFF informed ministers of the new outbreak and a further ten months elapsed before the government moved to have the threat assessed. MAFF also attempted to keep the nature of the disease to itself for as long as possible. When MAFF finally announced the existence of the new disease in October 1987, it did so in the Short Communications section of the *Veterinary Record* (journal of the British Veterinary Association). The government also kept tight control of information on BSE and journalists were given very little information. The very strictness of the official government line meant that those who disagreed with it had to find ways of communicating their ideas. So, willing alternative experts could easily be found and used as a balance to what little official information was being offered. This allowed the debate to widen and introduced a conflict at the level of science over the behaviour of the BSE agent and its potential consequences for animal and human life.

Scientific uncertainty

At the centre of this whole issue is the role of science. Had more been known about the BSE agent, clearer statements about diagnosis and treatment could have been made. But what became quickly clear was that, until scientific uncertainties about mad cow disease were cleared up, reassurances about the safety of British beef were not entirely convincing, and no firm resolution to the problem could be reached. The main debate has centred on the science of BSE and whether, through contamination via infected bovine products, it can be passed to humans. There has always been a theoretical risk that BSE could pass in this way. However, while many 'experts' on the subject have admitted to the possibility (however unlikely or remote they believed it to be), politicians did not, publicly at least. The message which was always highlighted by government was: 'There is no risk to humans.'

While no one believes that the government wanted to infect the population with a potentially fatal disease, decisions on BSE could not have been made based on pure science alone. Because of the lack of science, what should have been a scientific debate opened up into an economic and political one.

Controversy

BSE remained in the public sphere because controversy surrounded the subject. In April 1988 the government set up a committee (Southwood) to assess the significance of the new disease. The committee reported that:

> the risk of transmission of BSE to humans appears remote and it is unlikely that BSE will have any implications for human health.

But they also added:

> if our assessments of these likelihoods are incorrect, the implications would be extremely serious ... with the long incubation period of spongiform encephalopathies in humans, it may be a decade or more before complete reassurances can be given.

HMSO, 1989

In the government press conference held to highlight
the report it was stated:

> the report concludes that the risk of transmission of
> BSE to humans appears remote and it is therefore
> most unlikely that BSE will have any implications for
> human health.

BBC News, 27 February 1989

The Southwood committee had wanted 75 per
cent compensation for those farmers with infected cattle
(fearing they might sell them, send them to market
quickly, or destroy and bury them privately). But the
government disagreed, and the farmers had to settle for
50 per cent. In July 1988, John MacGregor, Minister of
Agriculture, stopped brains and offal being fed to cattle
and sheep. Inevitably, the next question to be asked (by
the DoH and opposition parties) was about human food.
While animals were no longer eating specified offals,
there was no such legislation for humans. Pre-clinical
BSE cattle were still going into the national food chain as
if they were healthy animals. Brains, spinal cord, spleen,
thymus, tonsils, intestines and bits of spinal tissue in
'mechanically recovered meat' were being used in a
variety of products such as burgers, meat pies, pâtés,
lasagne, soups, stock cubes and baby foods. In early
1989, the official government view was that the removal
of offals from human food was completely unnecessary.
By March 1989, MacGregor was asked to ban human
consumption of any organs known to harbour infectious
agents. In May of that year, Hugh Fraser, from the
Institute of Animal Health, and one of the most senior
researchers at the time, said on Radio 4's *Face the Facts*
that he no longer ate bovine offals, and that it would be

prudent if suspect tissues were removed from human consumption. This was finally done in November 1989.

Other factors ensured that BSE would remain a high-profile issue. There was already a well-developed interest in food safety because of salmonella and listeria which were high-profile public issues throughout 1988/9. By 1989, other countries began to be interested in the disease (Australia had already banned British beef cattle imports in July 1988). Germany, Italy and France banned British beef imports. The issue, in British terms, became political and economic. European countries claimed they were protecting public health. John Gummer (who had by this time been appointed Minister of Agriculture) treated this as powerful vested interests playing at protectionism. In Britain, local councils began banning British beef from the menus of 2,000 schools. Then the death of a domestic cat from a spongiform encephalopathy caused alarm, opening the debate on transmission between species and bringing the potential threat to humans a little closer to home. Early on in the crisis John Gummer took a close interest in the presentation of MAFF. He became the pre-eminent spokesman on BSE and Ministry vets were therefore not at the forefront of any public relations efforts. By 1990 BSE was the biggest story on the news. The government was forced into action. As part of a move to try to restore public confidence in beef they instituted a 'Beef is Safe' campaign. One of the most memorable aspects of the media campaign was Gummer's attempt at banishing 'mad cow hysteria' by feeding a beefburger to his young daughter. Surprisingly enough, it did not work, and concern mounted.

Media headlines – BSE

Yet the BSE story could not be sustained on a day-to-day level in news terms. Government inaction can cause uproar but that will die down when officials are seen to be doing something about it. This was clear when we see how BSE began to disappear from the media agenda once Britain had some success in stopping European bans on beef in 1990. While media coverage of BSE all but disappeared after 1990/1, the disease (as with salmonella levels) did not go away.

BSE: number of cases of infection in the UK against the number of articles in UK national newspapers (1986–96)

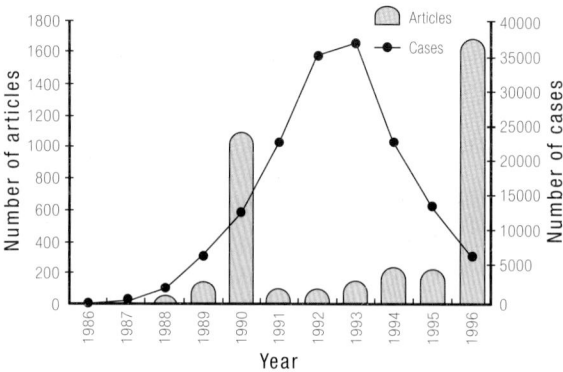

Although there had been a certain amount of media interest in the intervening years, it was not until March 1996 that a full-scale attack on this assessment of risk was heard. The fading interest had nothing to do with a change in MAFF's activity, nor any kind of scientific resolution, nor a decline in the spread of BSE. Rather, coverage reduced because there was a resolution of sorts on a political level. A compromise solution was instituted that reinstated beef imports to Europe so long as they were certified to come from BSE-free herds. However, the central issue of human transmission was not resolved by the European Community decision. In spite of, or perhaps because of, the outstanding scientific uncertainty, the decline in coverage towards the end of 1990 was sustained for the next five years, with only the occasional minor peak.

Main issues highlighted

- Government inaction and the power of the farming lobby to control policy decisions.
- Transmission to other species (animal).
- The lack of solid evidence either way about the safety of eating meat. For the government the decision about what to say related strongly to questions of public confidence and perceptions about levels of risk and what the risks were. In official government terms this translated into media statements such as 'British beef is safe' and 'there is no risk to human health'. For critics, it meant that there was a risk that eating beef was not safe, there was a 'potential risk', a 'theoretical risk', a 'low but significant risk'.
- The power of the European Community over Britain.

BSE retained the potential to re-emerge but required further scientific evidence or renewed official action. At this stage, MAFF's efforts to control the issue were actually quite effective. But also, because MAFF attempted to keep such tight control over information on BSE and CJD, alternative media sources were found, and 'experts' as such created. Behind the scenes, sources used by the media would be scientists, researchers, and organizations such as the British Veterinary Association. In this way questions which were not being asked at other levels could be addressed. The highlighting, for example, of conditions and practices within slaughterhouses changed the issue from whether bovine offals were being removed to how effectively or safely this was being done. An EHO document sent to MAFF in February 1990 had pointed out that poor practices were evident. They received no reply from the Ministry. It was only in 1995 (six years after implementation of policy in relation to slaughterhouse practices) that MAFF took steps to tighten controls on slaughterhouse practices. Had the media not brought research into poor hygiene and clear breaches of regulation into the open, work by, for example, the EHO might have gone unnoticed.

'It did help. We approached certain journalists and said, look we've found out that there are some disgracefully risky things going on in abattoirs, and something has to be done about it. Will you print it? The good ones … agreed. Now while that would have happened eventually, with government it is necessary to get the ball rolling, everything takes such a long time. But if there is public concern that can move things along … and with BSE the government were so paranoid about not being seen to be doing something that they reacted pretty damn quickly. It's not the ideal way of doing things, but when needs must.'
Member of the Institute of Environmental Health Officers, interviewed 1995

The general low level of media interest in Britain during 1991–5 was due, in part, to the feeling that BSE had exhausted its news value. There were also very

'Scientists continually said "we don't have the data, we need further research"... so we tended not to write about it ... It just doesn't make very good copy, to simply say "we don't know, we need further research", "we can't answer that". However honest that is, it doesn't play very well in terms of headlines.'
Broadsheet journalist, interviewed 1995

few new events to maintain a momentum of media concern. While a number of journalists remained intensely interested in BSE, they fell foul of editorial decision-making and the demands of news.

At the same time the lack of policy activity meant that editors lost interest in the subject because 'nothing was happening'. This reaction frustrated some journalists, because, as one broadsheet specialist pointed out: 'Of course that was the whole point, *nothing was happening* to destroy this thing; but in newspaper terms I wouldn't be given the space to say that every day or every week.' Simultaneously, MAFF's caution over what could be said in public minimized the chance that official sources would make controversial statements. For example, official experts who were taking precautions were not prepared to say that in public.

While clear pronouncements about safety were being made to the public, new cases of CJD had started to appear in 1994, when there were six, and continued in 1995. Ten cases had appeared in younger people (under 42 years). The most important aspect of them was that they were similar to each other both in clinical symptoms and in the pathological damage that appeared in the brain. John Pattison, Head of the Spongiform Encephalopathy Advisory Committee (SEAC), suggested that projected cases of BSE in humans, calculated on current information, could represent a major public health problem.

Under Pattison's headship SEAC decided that the news had to be made public.

The announcement led to an explosion of media coverage, even exceeding the previous peak of interest in 1990. While public health interests were finally brought into play, government failure to deal adequately with BSE earlier was all the stronger and European interventions were dramatically strengthened in 1996 with demands for a worldwide ban on British beef and a major culling policy.

'I couldn't believe it. They were actually going to do it. I mean this was huge, absolutely huge. I can just imagine the utter panic in MAFF. For another department in their own government to come out and say the complete opposite to what they'd been saying for eleven years – God, it was certainly a brave move. But it couldn't be stopped. Too many chinks in the "there is no risk" armour had been pierced. It was all so inevitable really, and so bloody tragic. Hogg's [Douglas Hogg, the Minister of Agriculture] reaction was pathetic but predictable, the "it's not fair" number. MAFF had certainly blown it this time, and you could feel the shock waves reverberating around everyone involved with this thing from government to sausage makers ... it was the end of the line, a link had been found. The media were there to glory in their misery ... they must have thought it was Christmas, and we thought this really was going to be a nightmare ...'
Scientist, interviewed 1996

Changes in government action

Going public with information on a new strain of CJD had changed the nature of the BSE debate. Health interests had been brought into play. While SEAC made recommendations that the 'risk' to humans from food would probably be small if there were better controls on offals, and more rigorous enforcement of those controls, Prime Minster John Major was saying that beef was 'entirely safe' and that this 'had been confirmed by British scientists' (*PM*, 23 April 1996).

European action

European intervention was what brought the disease to the forefront in 1990, 1992 and again in 1996. European countries claimed they were protecting public health. In

1990 John Gummer treated this as powerful vested interests playing at protectionism, aided by 'media hype and sensationalism'. He issued what could be described as a call to arms, asking that we all, 'including the BBC, ITN and others', refuse to let the European Community control Britain. Yet it took until 1999 for all of the bans on exporting British beef to be lifted as countries demanded ever stronger assurances that Britain was doing enough to eradicate the disease.

Conclusion

There is a sense in which lessons have been learned from BSE. Government is now seen to be at some level more open. For example, data from the BSE Inquiry, set up to investigate how it happened, is accessible to the public. Confidence in British beef is seen to be returning. But all of this has come at a cost. While the number of BSE-infected cattle is down to below one hundred per week and the disease may well be eradicated, it is estimated to have cost at least £4.6 billion, as well as the cost of businesses and jobs from the beef-production chain to farmers and slaughterhouses, retailers, and restaurants. In addition, to 30 June 1999, the number of definite and probable cases of new variant Creutzfeldt-Jakob disease (nvCJD) is 43 (Creutzfeldt-Jakob Disease Surveillance Unit figures). In terms of long-term damage though, the cost of the BSE crisis is probably much more. Because, as with salmonella, just as the crisis around BSE seemed to be over, another food issue began to become much more high profile – genetically modified food.

Genetically
Modified Food

Biotechnology is a rather confusing umbrella term for a wide range of scientific techniques that make use of living cells and organisms to produce food and organisms. It covers everything from traditional breeding and cheese production to modern genetic engineering. *Traditional biotechnology* techniques, such as the fermentation of yeast and the use of lactic acid bacteria to make yoghurt, have been around for years. Other new and powerful techniques fall into the *modern biotechnology* category. Now scientists are able to transfer genetic material between organisms in a way that cannot be achieved by natural methods of mating or cross-breeding. Other terms used for this process include *genetic engineering*, *modification* and *manipulation*. The organisms created in this way are called *genetically modified organisms* (GMOs). When these are foodstuffs they are called *novel foods*.

Genetically Modified Foods: Magic Solution or Hidden Menace? Consumers International, Briefing paper, No. 8, November 1997

GM food and crops have begun receiving increasing political and media attention in Britain.

So what is all the fuss about? Is the use of this new technology in relation to the production of food just another 'scare', or are there relevant concerns relating to the uses of this science in connection with what we eat?

Genetic modification (GM) and the use of genetically modified crops are now being introduced in a context which has been culturally transformed by the BSE experience. Formulating policy on a technology over which there are still considerable uncertainties (scientific, ethical and political) demands a risk culture which does not replicate previous mistakes. There are, however, signs that some of the errors, false reassurances and commercial complicity evidenced during the BSE crisis are compromising a precautionary approach to GMOs. Genetic modification and genetically modified food crops pose analogous risks to those posed by BSE:

- The link between BSE and CJD took a long time to show and was established only after active monitoring. Possible harm from genetically modified foods may take even longer to detect and establish.
- The effects of GM could be serious and irreversible.
- There is considerable scientific uncertainty over the potential impacts of GM.

From BSE to Genetically Modified Organisms: Science, Uncertainty and the Precautionary Principle by J. Sheppard, Greenpeace Report, July 1997

The high profile of genetically modified foods has occurred for a number of reasons. Firstly, they are here – the crops are being tested and the products are on supermarket shelves (for now at least). Secondly, there have been growing and concerted attempts by pressure groups (both environmental and consumer) to get

In relation to genetically modified food products, the industry line has been dominated by issues around these new foods leading to lower prices, better quality and a longer shelf life. When interviewed or quoted, industry officials on the whole stress that safety is not the prime issue but communication with the public to reassure them that there are no risks associated with eating these products.

The second major discourse in this area is that expounded by those attempting to curb advances of genetically modified products. This discourse has a particularly wide remit which suggests that there are important implications for health, the environment, ethics and the economy. The main argument is that consumers have the right to information about the safety of the technologies and specifically about labelling and regulation of products being sold. Concerns centre on the speed with which the technologies are progressing without 'proper' regulation and the perception that modern biotechnology is in commercial hands and therefore public accountability will take second place to financial imperatives.

The main issues discussed

Since 1996 pressure groups have been more successful in using, amongst other things, the media to force issues onto the political agenda. The mass media have been used in some circumstances to serve as one avenue for public information and political/policy leverage. Mass media reporting generally reflects the level of coordination and centralized information sources in any given field. In the face of official silence and lack of coordination, journalists have contacted

Although the debate surrounding genetically modified organisms has focused mainly upon the risks of the technology, we must not lose sight of its huge potential benefits in areas of food supply, food quality, nutrition and health. When one considers that the world population is expected to reach 8 billion by 2020, it is clear that new approaches will be needed in addition to the continued improvement of existing methods of crop and animal husbandry and food processing in order to feed such a burgeoning population.

Genetically Modified Foods – Royal Society Calls for a Rational Debate, Royal Society statement, 13 August 1998

We're excited about the potential for genetically modified food to contribute to a better environment and a sustainable, plentiful, and healthy food supply. We recognise, however, that many consumers have genuine concerns about food biotechnology and its impact on their families.

Monsanto web site: *http://www.monsanto.co.uk*

scientists, pressure groups and research institutes directly. Yet in 1998 scientists interviewed emphasized that they increasingly perceived a need to communicate with the media, not least because of the growing influence of pressure groups in the genetically modified technologies debate. Journalists also reported growing source activity to discuss the implications of research and the introduction of new products. The progress of the science has generated changes in mass media coverage and wider questions are being asked within mass media formats. The development of the debate in this way has impacted at different levels. For example, it seems that the companies producing GM products did not sufficiently take into account 'negative' media coverage around consumer groups and EU concerns over maize and soya which had been building up in newspapers since July 1996.

Many commentators, especially those sympathetic to the biotechnology industry, have been keen to portray the GE [genetically engineered] food crisis as yet another in a long line of British 'food scares', exaggerated crises whipped up by the media ... there is undoubtedly some truth in the 'food scare' analysis, but there is also a substantial amount of self comfort. Much of the concern is undoubtedly rather superficial, and is based on over-excited and inaccurate media reports. The British media was clearly looking for an issue to embarrass the government with, and, for once, the government handled public opinion very poorly. But those who wish to dismiss public concern should remember that it only flares up at particular moments because of an underlying, deep-seated, and justifiable concern about how our food is produced and what it is doing to us. Put simply, people do not want their food mucked around with, especially when they see no clear benefits to themselves.
GenEthics News: Genetic Engineering, Ethics and the Environment, Issue 28/29, Spring/Summer 1999

In general there is a sense in which mass media formats have failed to address some of the fundamental and more complex questions present in contemporary debates (it is easier to get much more information via the Internet, for example). It is obvious that media coverage of genetically modified food and crops is selective, but at the same time the mass media are a useful tool in helping to get issues onto the political and public agendas.

This increase has been due primarily to the appearance of GM products on supermarket shelves and to the legal and agricultural changes which have occurred because of GM crops, and because there has been a growing debate in general on food issues such as BSE and E. coli. As has already been suggested, BSE has altered the nature of coverage in newspapers in general. While there were a number of papers which were questioning the risks and benefits associated with GM food and crops before March 1996 (most notably *The Guardian, Independent* and *Observer*), after the announcement of a potential link between BSE and CJD, the vast majority of feature coverage has centred on the uncertainties associated with these technologies and problems perceived with a lack of proper regulation.

In the commercial sphere, there is a dynamic and potentially profitable innovation in GMOs on a mounting international scale. The first GMO commercial consumer products are now being sanctioned and sold in the UK, and pressure for the introduction of more may now be expected to intensify.

In the lay public sphere, there is little familiarity with GMO technology, but well-grounded, if largely latent, anxieties about the implications of the technology itself, and about the limitations of current regulatory arrangements for addressing such arrangements. In these circumstances, a few non-governmental organisations, rather than the designated official bodies, are tending to be perceived as, effectively, the watchdogs on society's behalf. Moreover, few significant compensating benefits to society itself are felt currently to arise from exploitation of the technology, which is perceived to be driven largely by straightforward commercial considerations.

Uncertain World: Genetically Modified Organisms, Food and Public Attitudes in Britain, Centre for the Study of Environmental Change report, 1997

Debates around genetically modified food and crops have been given space because the subject has been contentious. So, while pressure groups have pursued media attention in their campaigns for safety measures, consumer protection and choice, experts have complained of media 'scare-mongering', industry and government bodies have attempted to maintain public confidence, and journalists have described the attractions of controversy. There has been a great deal of concern from some quarters that, while industry may see financial gain and no risks from the new technologies, the products are being forced on a public who have not been asked if they want them, and to a large extent do not understand what the science is all about.

Labelling, choice and health

Labelling is at the heart of the debate about choice. Genetically modified products have been on British supermarket shelves since 1996. While the first product, a tomato purée produced by Zeneca, was labelled, another company, Monsanto, then introduced unlabelled genetically modified soya to the European market. This produced an outcry from European groups who claimed that consumers needed to be given the choice to know whether they were eating food that had genetically modified ingredients.

In March 1998 Iceland announced that it would remove genetically modified soya from its stores. It was clear that Monsanto had underestimated the opposition to these products in Britain and they took out full-page adverts in the national press (June 1998) to reassure the public about the safety of their products. But public confidence in these products has continued to fall sharply as the debate about their safety continued and widened. Prince Charles entered the debate by commenting on the potential problems of growing genetically engineered crops in June 1998 (his views on this issue having been made public from as early as 1995).

> Mainstream consumers as well as environmental organisations have demanded comprehensive labelling and segregation of GM foods. Such demands have several sources: resentment at being denied a choice; distrust of official safety judgements; and the consumer choice as an indirect means to 'vote' on agricultural methods of producing food. Thus public trust depends upon clear labelling of any products which may contain GM ingredients.
>
> 'What science? UK controversy over genetically modified crops and food' by L. Levidow, in R. Miettinen (ed.), *Biotechnology and Public Understanding of Science*, publication of the Academy of Finland, 1998

The introduction of labelling laws in relation to genetically modified food was finally agreed in 1998. But this did not end the debate. In 1999 political and mass media interest continued to be stimulated because of genetically modified crop trials and individuals' and organizations' attempts to sabotage them, scientists coming out both for and against genetically modified products, and pressure from a number of consumer, health and environmental organizations which resulted in supermarkets, retailers and caterers announcing that they would not use genetically modified ingredients in their products.

Given the high profile of the genetic modification debate, the central question remains – are these products risky for humans? The answer is that no one yet knows. No one knows whether consuming genetically modified soya or tomatoes will affect human health or how testing genetically modified crops in fields will affect the environment (or even non-GM crops planted close to them). The main point being made by those critical of the speed with which this new technology is being used, is that there are too many uncertainties for us to accept it unquestioningly.

There is no evidence that any of the genetically modified foods on sale at the moment pose any risk to the health of people eating them. But that is not the same as saying they can be guaranteed 100% safe. It is clear that we don't yet have enough evidence. The government's Chief Scientific Adviser, Sir Robert May, says, 'More research needs to be done. We don't have all the answers. But in the meantime we shouldn't reject genetically modified crops and food out of hand.' Sceptics may not find this reassuring. Many will remember how Sir Robert's former counterpart, Sir Donald Acheson, the Chief Medical Officer at the Department of Health, ressured the public over BSE in 1990. He said then that there was 'no risk' associated with eating British beef. In 1998 he admitted, 'I should not have said that, because the advice of my [expert] groups was that there was a remote risk, not no risk.'

GM Free: A Shopper's Guide to Genetically Modified Food by S. Dibb and T. Lobstein, London, Virgin Publishing Ltd, 1999

Knowing the history of food safety in Britain it is perhaps understandable that people are concerned about a technology they have no experience of, and potentially do not trust. If genetically modified foods turn out to be safe all the more good, but it is clear that until this is proven, reservations about using the products will remain. One of many surveys carried out in 1999 claimed that 68 per cent of the people questioned were concerned about eating genetically modified food and more 75 per cent said that, until more research has been carried out, there should be a ban on genetically modified products (NOP survey for *Independent on Sunday*, 21 February 1999).

While Monsanto has since publicly stated that it will not pull out of Britain it is clear that large companies do still have problems if they want to sell their products. While some people may remain unconcerned about the potential risks from genetic modification, surely no one would disagree that keeping an eye on how technologies develop is no bad thing in relation to food safety and consumer confidence.

Conclusion

Is our food poisoning us? The answer to that question seems to be dependent on whom you ask. The true incidence of food poisoning is said to be vastly under-reported with perhaps as few as one in twenty cases being recognized. The industrialization of food production over the last twenty or thirty years has meant that food has become a complex global business which means that more things can go wrong: look at what happened when cows were given feed containing other animals because it was economically cheaper, or the introduction of new technologies such as genetic modification – the risks from which will only become visible in the future. What about the presence of new bugs such as E. coli which are not properly understood as yet, and the fact that bacteria are becoming harder to treat as they become more resistant to antibiotics.

What is clear is that there are a number of risks associated with food which we have to take seriously. There are a widening number of issues which people now have to deal with in relation to food. Proper checks on hygiene, cooking and risks of infection from cross-contamination need to be taken seriously at all levels of the food production chain from the farm to the home.

In April 2000, over three years after it was promised by the Labour government, the Food Standards Agency came into being. Where food safety was once the responsibility of the Ministry of Agriculture, the setting up of the Food Standards Agency is being seen as a radical change from what has gone before. The objective of this independent agency is to clean up the country's food supply as well as the climate of confusion and suspicion about the safety of our food. The agency aims to do this by, for example, putting in place tougher meat hygiene measures, having more controls on BSE, and attempting to cut the rate of salmonella in chickens by half within five years. They have also claimed that they will be more open, will have meetings in public, will publish evidence and advice to government ministers and will 'name and shame' companies which break the rules. By being vigorous both with government and the food industry the agency claims that it will put the consumer first. It remains to be seen how independent the agency will be, as food is one of the biggest manufacturing sectors in the British economy. The Food Standards Agency will undoubtedly come up against vested interests from the food industry in its pursuit of more comprehensive food safety legislation. But its success will undoubtedly lie in whether it can gain the trust of the public and manage to put public health at the top of the political agenda.

So how can this new independent agency gain public trust after so many disasters in relation to food safety in recent British history? Apart from tightening up food hygiene legislation and food production standards from the factories and farms, the agency should attempt to understand the people better that they claim to be representing – the public. It has already been criticized for not having enough consumer representation. If this is the case then there will undoubtedly be problems. If there is no proper consumer power base then food safety in relation to consumers' perception of safety will not change radically. Historically, within political and industrial spheres, it has commonly been the case that the mass media are blamed for helping to cause food scares while the public are blamed for seemingly reacting to 'scare' information in an 'irrational' way. Words commonly used to express public reactions tend to be 'alarm', 'fear', 'confusion' or 'panic'.

But there are a number of problems with this notion. The 'public' is not a single homogeneous mass who will act identically in any given situation. There are as many different reactions to issues as there are issues raised. This is probably because people tend to get information from a number of different sources. If you ask someone where they found out about a specific issue the variety of answers may include television, newspapers, radio, magazines, leaflets, advertising, health education, doctors, family, friends or from personal experience. The source of the information is used to judge the validity of both old and new information which may appear in the media or elsewhere. What may also be relevant are that age, gender, income, class, personal experience and national and cultural identity can be important in determining how people will assess information.

We have to ask when these 'scares' do arise, who is actually 'alarmed', 'confused' or 'panicked'. Certainly there will be levels of public concern, but at the same time we must look at who has the most to lose by food safety issues being highlighted. Members of the public may choose to ignore food safety information or to stop eating a particular product. But it is the government, food industry, farming community and catering facilities who have the most to lose in terms of costs and credibility. To simply blame the media for reporting or the public for supposedly 'panicking' assumes that the so-called 'scares' are at some level not real. But there *was* a rise in levels of salmonella poisoning and herds *have* been infected with BSE (and humans potentially with CJD). It would not be advisable for any agency attempting to win the trust of the public to ignore the complex ways that people tend to make decisions about what they eat.

Food safety issues do tend to be seen, in general, as issues which have a certain life span – probably because of the way they appear in the mass media (huge amounts of coverage which disappear once something is seen to have been done). There may be a great deal of concern when they are highlighted but people will go back to normal practices once the issue has retreated from the news. This may be the case for salmonella in eggs: think how concerned you are about eating an egg at the moment, even though levels of the infection are higher than they were in 1988. It was also the case with BSE following the slump in the public debate from 1991 until 1996. The changes brought about since 1996 have not only impacted at government or industry level, but also to some extent changed how people perceive risk information in relation to food. And it may also be the case that, because of the impact of BSE in Britain, the debate around genetically modified food has followed the course it has done. The marked rise in the sale of organic produce, up by at least one third in 1999 from the previous year, may indicate a changing attitude to what consumers see as being 'safe'.

At this time there is a lot of information which can be accessed by those wishing to get a more balanced view of what any given problem is about. As consumers we have the right to expect safe food, and in those cases where there may be a risk associated with a certain product, to be told truthfully what the risks are. Consumers do not need to be treated as though they are 'stupid' or 'irrational', not able to deal with the uncertainties arising from food safety issues. If we are given all of the available information, most people will come to a decision about whether they believe there is a risk associated with food or not. We have to be given that choice, and this can only be done if potential problems associated with food are aired before consumers in order that they can make their own minds up. As we have seen from the BSE crisis, keeping information out of the public domain, or making reassurances of safety when there is no firm scientific proof, can backfire spectacularly.

Further Reading

Eat Your Genes: How Genetically Modified Food is Entering Your Diet by S. Nottingham, Nottingham, Zed Books, 1998.

Fatal Legacy: BSE, the Search for the Truth by S. Dealler, London, Corgi, 1996.

Food, Health and Identity by P. Caplan, London, Routledge, 1997.

Food Scares in the Media by D. Miller and J. Reilly, Glasgow, Glasgow University Media Group, 1994.

From BSE to Genetically Modified Organisms: Science, Uncertainty and the Precautionary Principle by J. Sheppard, Greenpeace Briefing Paper, July 1997.

GM Free: A Shopper's Guide to Genetically Modified Food by S. Dibb and T. Lobstein, London, Virgin Ltd, 1999.

The Food We Eat by J. Blythman, England, Penguin, 1998.

The Kind Food Guide by A. Eyton, England, Penguin, 1991.

The Nation's Diet: The Social Science of Food Choice by A. Murcott (ed.), London, Longman, 1998.

The Politics of Food by G. Cannon, London, Century, 1987.